YOGA FOR

STRESS

RELIEF

CALM YOUR MIND, BODY AND SPIRIT

Carise Jordan

You cannot always control what goes on outside,
But you can always control what goes on inside.

Table of Contents

INTRODUCTION

Stress is a Sudden Biological Change. It has become the curse of the 21st century and is a silent killer in the modern world. Stress is the greatest danger to the information era. Stress is the priceless poison for human life in the universe. It can disturb any one's physical, mental, emotional and behavioral balance. Stress can damage different parts of human body from muscles and tissues to organs and blood vessels. It can speed up pulse rate and respiration. It can raise blood pressure and body temperature. It can also interfere with the body metabolism, digestion, appetite, sleep, sexuality and even fertility. Occupational stress includes the environmental factors or stressors such as work overload, role ambiguity, role conflict and poor working conditions associated with a particular job.

There are three stages a person goes through while suffering from stress.

ALARM STAGE

This stage experiences an over acting of the sympathetic nervous system wherein adrenaline and cortisol increase and blood flows away from the brain to the muscles. As a result, dendrites shrink back in the brain to moderate the flow of information, slowing or closing down the nonessential body functions. The whole body starts preparing itself to fight against the reason of stress. The fear, excitement or pressure is evident on the sufferer's face.

RESISTANCE STAGE

In this stage, the body keeps making continuous efforts to cope with stress and therefore feels run down and the person starts feeling irritated, over reacts to minor situations and gets mentally and physically weak. Psychological, physical and behavioral changes are also clearly visible.

EXHAUSTION STAGE

If a student is preparing for his exam and despite of every possible effort, he is not able to relate to his studies, he is bound to get stressed. The stress could reach a height where he/she may feel completely exhausted and helpless to the extent of committing suicide.

This is the exhaustion stage. This stage is further divided into two phases: The nature of stress is broadly of two types- Eustress (Positive stress, Distress (Negative stress).

SIGNS AND SYMPTOMS OF STRESS

If exposure to stressors continues for a longer period of time, chronic health problems can develop, such as:

Psychological and emotional

Feeling heroic, invulnerable, euphoric, Denial, Anxiety and fear,

Worry about safety of self and others, Anger, Irritability, Restlessness, Sadness, grief, depression, moodiness, Distressing dreams, Guilt or "survivor guilt", Feeling overwhelmed, hopeless, Feeling isolated, lost, or abandoned, Apathy, Identification with survivors.

Cognitive

Memory problems, Disorientation, Confusion, Slowness of thinking and comprehension, Difficulty calculating, setting priorities, making decisions, Poor concentration, Limited attention span, Loss of objectivity, Unable to stop thinking about the disaster, Blaming

Behavioral

Change in activity, Decreased efficiency and effectiveness, Difficulty communicating, Increased sense of humor, Outbursts of anger, fre□uent arguments, Inability to rest or "letdown", Change in eating habits, Change in sleeping patterns, Change in patterns of intimacy, sexuality, Change in job performance,Periods of crying, Increased use of alcohol, tobacco, or drugs, Social withdrawal, silence, Vigilance about safety or environment, Avoidance of activities or places that trigger memories, Proneness to accidents

Physical

Increased heartbeat, respiration, Increased blood pressure, Upset stomach, nausea, diarrhea, Change in appetite, weight loss or gain,

Sweating or chills, Tremors (hands, lips), Muscle twitching, "Muffled" hearing, Tunnel vision, Feeling uncoordinated, Headaches, Soreness in muscles, Lower back pain, Feeling a "lump in the throat", Exaggerated startle reaction, Fatigue, Menstrual cycle changes, Change in sexual desire, Decreased resistance to infection, Flare-up of allergies and arthritis, Hair loss

Yoga for Stress Relief

Yoga is most Recognized form of Exercise, Stretching, Aerobic exercise and Meditation. The definition of yoga is "to yoke or joint together" it integrates the mind and body focusing on balance posture, deep breathing, stretching and relaxation. Yoga evolved from of the Hindu, Jaina, and Buddhist religious traditions in India. Yoga alters stress response and person's attitude, towards stress along with improving self confidence, increasing one's sense of well being, and creating a feeling of relaxation and calmness.

CHAPTER ONE

ORIGIN OF YOGA

Nobody knows precisely when Yoga started, however it absolutely originates before recorded history. Yoga positions portrayed by stone carving have been obtain in archeological destinations in the Indus Valley going back 5,000 years or more. There is a typical misguided judgment that Yoga is established in Hinduism; unexpectedly, Hinduism's religious structures developed much later and fused a portion of the acts of Yoga. (Different religions all through the world have likewise joined practices and thoughts identified with Yoga.)

The convention of Yoga has dependably been passed on independently from educator to understudy through oral instructing and reasonable exhibition. The formal strategies that are currently known as Yoga seem to be, hence, in light of the aggregate encounters of numerous people over numerous of great years. The specific way in which the systems are educated and rehearsed today relies upon the methodology went down in the line of educators supporting the individual expert.

One of the soonest messages doing with Yoga was gathered by a researcher named Patanjali, who set down the most predominant Yoga speculations and practices of his time in a book he called Yoga Sutras ("Yoga Aphorisms") as ahead of schedule as the first or second century B.C. then again as late as the fifth century A.D. (Unknown exact dates). The framework that he expounded on is known as "Ashtanga Yoga," or the eight limbs of Yoga, and this is what is for the most part alluded to today as Classical Yoga. Most present followers rehearse some variety of Patanjali's framework.

The eight stages of Classical Yoga are:

➤ **Yama**, signifying "limitation" — abstaining from viciousness, lying, taking, easygoing sex, and storing;

➤ **Niyama**, signifying "recognition" — virtue, happiness, resilience, study, and recognition;

➤ **Asana**, physical activities;

➤ **Pranayama**, breathing methods;

➤ **Pratyahara,** readiness for reflection, portrayed as "withdrawal of the brain from the faculties";

➤ **Dharana,** fixation, having the capacity to hold the psyche on one item for a predetermined time;

➤ **Dhyana,** contemplation, the capacity to concentrate on one thing (or nothing) inconclusively;

> **Samadhi,** ingestion, or acknowledgment of the vital way of the self.

Modern Western Yoga classes widely concentrate on the third, fourth, and fifth steps. Yoga most likely touched base in the United States in the late 1800s, yet it didn't turn out to be broadly known until the 1960s, as a feature of the young society's developing enthusiasm for anything Eastern. As more got to be thought about the advantageous impacts of Yoga, it picked up acknowledgment and admiration as a profitable strategy for aiding in the administration of anxiety and enhancing wellbeing and prosperity. Numerous doctors now prescribe Yoga practice to patients at danger for coronary illness, and also those with back torment, joint inflammation, melancholy, and other interminable conditions.

WHAT IS YOGA?

Many of us have practiced Yoga for years, yet if someone asks us about a definition of what Yoga is, we would be hard pressed to give an answer. As many other important products of ancient Indian culture, Yoga isn't clearly defined and systematised like the scientific disciplines of the West. I will try to give a personal contribution to this subject; it is not a clear, simple definition I'm looking for, but rather an unveiling of the essence of this amazing science.

Modern definitions of Yoga.

Even though there aren't, in modern times, such famous definition as Patañjali's, it's still possible to identify some general approaches to Yoga.

Yoga as Fitness.

The main focus is placed on the practice of asanas (postures), and on the perfection of alignment. The therapeutic effects of each posture are sometimes studied in depth, so that a personalised practice can be devised, in order to address specific health conditions. In other styles of Yoga, the emphasis is on a powerful, dynamic practice that acts more as a prevention than a cure: which constantly stimulating energetic system and attaining a state of permanent physical balance and health.

Yoga as Meditation.

Another modern interpretation sees Yoga as primarily a meditation techni☐ue. Here, the focus is on calming and stabilising the mind, through the use of asanas, pranayama (breath control), as well as mental concentration techni☐ues. This interpretation usually do not give so much importance to alignment in the postures, or to the physical benefits of Yoga; instead, the body is used as a tool to access one own's mind and gain more control over it.

Yoga as Union.

Some practitioners and schools understand Yoga as a process of union between one's own internal world (sometimes called the "Microcosm") and the Universe (the "Macrocosm"), Nature, or God. This interpretation are very focused on Bhakti (devotional) practices, such as Mantra chanting, rituals, and so on. The practice of postures, breathing exercises, and other techni☐ues is seen as a tool to facilitate the union, or dissolution, of the individual Self into a higher, superior entity. The positive conse☐uences on health, as well as the mental concentration that can be attained through the practice of Yoga, are seen as secondary effects, although beneficial.

Yoga as Evolution.

Yoga is a practical philosophical system whose objective is the physical, mental and spiritual evolution of the human being.

YOGA HELPS REDUCE STRESS

➢ Yoga uses slow and deep belly breaths to lower your body's levels of the stress hormone cortisol.

➢ Yoga encourages people to practice "mindfulness," which can help combat stress over the long-term.

➢ Non-impact moves help get the stress-relieving benefits of physical exercise.

When you're stressed to the max, climbing onto the yoga mat might not be your first move. But for some, it could be a smart one. Stress can contribute to headaches, and taking steps to reduce stress may help some people avoid them.

It Deepens Your Breathing

There's a reason people say, "take a deep breath." Deep breathing literally slows your sympathetic nervous system, which acts a lot like a gas pedal for your body. Yoga uses slow and most importantly, deep belly breaths to lower your body's levels of the stress hormone cortisol as well as supply your brain with more of the oxygen it needs to work at its best. The result: You're calmer and better able to solve the problems causing you stress.

It Teaches Mindfulness

When people are stressed, it could be because they're dwelling on the past or worrying about the future. Yoga, however, encourages people to pay attention to their feelings in the present moment, a skill often termed "mindfulness." Practicing mindfulness techniques within your yoga practice and then implementing them throughout the day can help combat stress over the long-term.

It Improves Sleep

Stress and sleep (or rather a lack thereof) is a vicious cycle. Stress can throw off your sleep, which, in turn, makes you even more stressed. Yoga can help break the cycle.

It Gets You Moving

Exercise is becoming increasingly popular among the medical community as a treatment for down-in-the-dumps symptoms such as stress and anxiety. However, high-intensity exercise can temporarily increase your cortisol levels, which may put your body (and perhaps even your mind) under additional stress, Gentle forms of yoga, however, use non-impact moves to help get the stress-relieving benefits of physical exercise without triggering the release of stress-related hormones.

YOGA FOOD TIPS AND ADVICES FOR GOOD HEALTH

- ➢ Eat four times each day at four hour interims.
- ➢ Never try to skip breakfast, it is the most imperative dinner of the day.
- ➢ Never try to drink water with your feast – take water 30 minutes before a meal.
- ➢ When you eat a meal, your stomach ought to be 1/2 loaded with nourishment, ¼ with water (taking 30 minutes before) and ¼ ought to be vacant for appropriate absorption.
- ➢ Eat sustenance that is naturally cooked.
- ➢ Never try to gorge or eat too less.
- ➢ Nourishment ought to be delicious and simple to process.
- ➢ Nourishment ought to be eaten with focus and in a ☐uiet domain.

BENEFITS OF YOGA FOR THE MIND, BODY AND SPIRIT

➢ **All-round wellness.** You are genuinely solid when you are physically fit as well as rationally and candidly adjusted. As Sri Ravi Shankar puts it, "Wellbeing is not an insignificant nonattendance of malady. It is a dynamic articulation of life – as far as how happy, adoring and eager you are." This is the place yoga helps: stances, pranayama (breathing systems) and contemplation are a comprehensive wellness bundle.

➢ **Weight loss.** Yoga is advantageous. Sun Salutations and Kapal Bhati pranayama are some ways to help reducing in weight with yoga. Moreover, with regular rehearse of yoga, we tend to become more sensitive to the kind of food our body asks for and when. This also help keep a check on your weight.

➢ **Stress help.** Little minutes of yoga amid the day can be of incredible approach to decreases stress that aggregates every day - both the body and brain. Yoga stances, pranayama and meditation are one of a kind procedures to alleviation stress.

➢ **Inner peace.** We love to visit ☐uiet, tran☐uil spots, rich in normal excellence. Little do we understand that peace can be discovered right inside us and we can take a smaller than usual get-away to experience this at whatever time of the day!

Advantage from a little occasion each day with yoga and reflection. Yoga is likewise one of the most ideal approaches to quiet an exasperates mind.

➢ **Improved insusceptibility.** Our framework is a consistent mix of the body, psyche and soul. An anomaly in the body influences the psyche and comparably offensiveness or fretfulness in the brain can show as a disease in the body. Yoga postures knead organs and strengthen muscles; breathing procedures and meditation discharge push and enhance insusceptibility.

➢ **Better connections.** Yoga can even enhance your association with your life partner, guardians, companions or friends and family! A psyche that is casual, upbeat and mollified is better ready to manage delicate relationship matters. Yoga and meditation chip away at keeping the brain cheerful and serene; advantage from the reinforced exceptional bond you impart to individuals near you.

CHAPTER TWO

CHAKRAS

The term chakra comes from **Sanskrit** the ancient, sacred language of India and means *"spinning wheel"*. It refers to the ever turning energy centers that are a part of your subtle or energetic body. Yogis and clairvoyant seers (people who can see energy and auras) describe chakras as spinning fans, lotus flowers, or suns of light stacked along the body.

While chakras are not physical, they do correspond to specific locations, organs, hormones and activities of the body. They also influence and are influenced by your thoughts, feelings and life areas. Their function is to process life force energy (known as prana or chi) to bring about holistic wellness.

Although there are thousands of chakras all over the body, yoga and healing practices focus mainly on the seven major chakras. Optimizing these major chakras automatically enhances the functioning of all other (smaller) chakras.

The seven main chakras:

First Chakra: Root

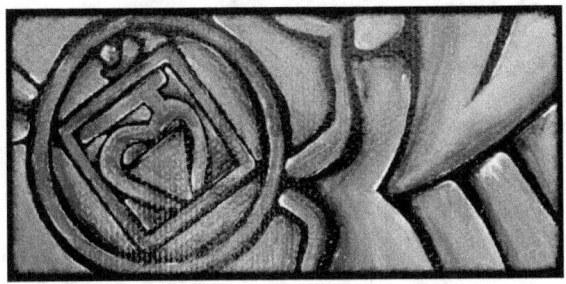

Sanskrit Name: Muladhara (meaning support)

Colour: Red

Location: Base of spine

Corresponding areas: Survival, physical grounding, sustenance and abundance, feeling safe, secure and supported, having basic needs met.

Affirmation: I am safe, secure and supported in all ways.

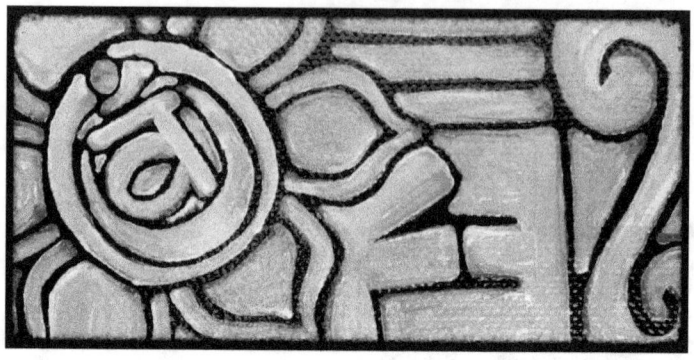

Sanskrit Name: Svadhisthana (meaning sweetness)

Colour: Orange

Location: Below the naval/belly button

Corresponding areas: Pleasure, passion, sexuality, fertility, creativity, desires, appetites and cravings, enjoying life in physical ways, sense of deserving and being worthy

Affirmation: I am perfectly balanced in all my desires, and I live my life with great joy.

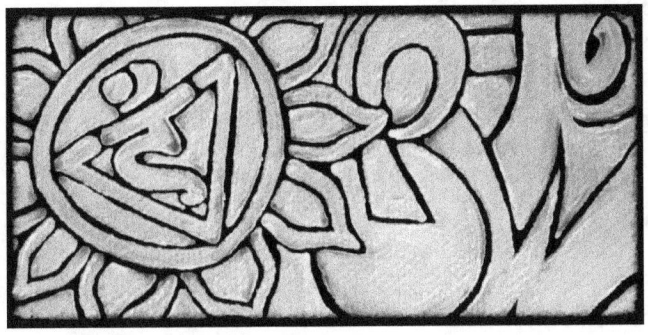

Sanskrit Name: Manipura (meaning sparkling jewel)

Colour: Yellow

Location: Center of stomach, above the naval

Corresponding areas: Personal power, self-worth, self-esteem, self-respect, self-control, strength of will, energy, spontaneity, courage, confidence, resilience, purpose

Affirmation: I have the power in my life, and I use it to achieve my dreams and do what honours me.

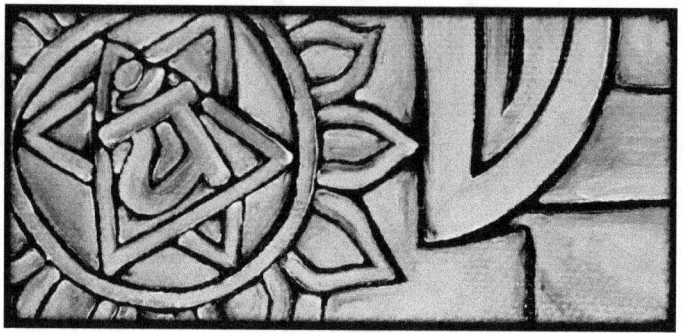

Sanskrit Name: Anahata (meaning flawless)

Colour: Green

Location: Center of chest

Corresponding areas: Love, compassion, forgiveness, empathy, humanity, self-acceptance,

clairsentience (clear/intuitive feeling), balance, healthy relationships

Affirmation: I am a being of love and I radiate this love to myself and everyone.

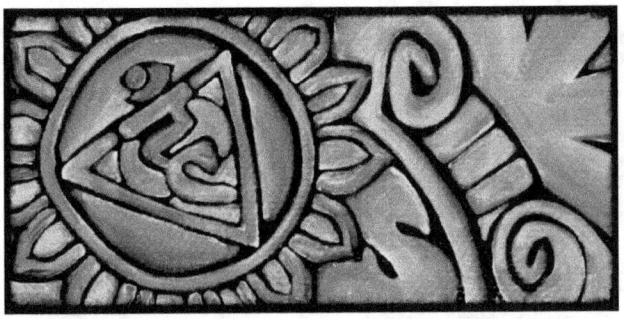

Sanskrit Name: Vissudha (meaning purity)

Colour: Light blue

Location: Center of throat

Corresponding areas: Truth, communication, creative and artistic expression, inspiration

Affirmation: I speak my truth with love and express myself with grace and integrity.

Sixth Chakra: Third Eye

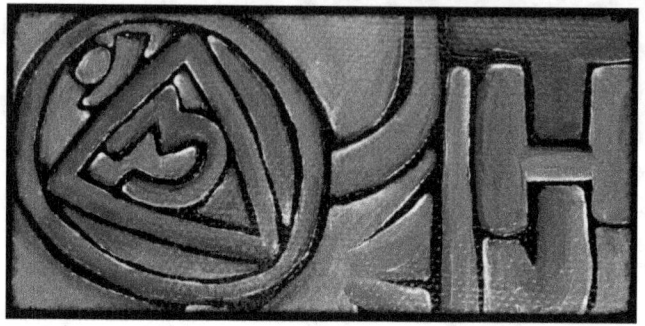

Sanskrit Name: Ajna (meaning awareness, perception)

Colour: Indigo, dark blue with some deep purple

Location: Middle of forehead

Corresponding areas: Intuition, perception, visualization, imagination, clairvoyance (clear seeing), accurate interpretation, wisdom, knowledge, truth, intelligence

Affirmation: I see the truth in all situations and let my inner wisdom guide me.

Seventh Chakra: Crown

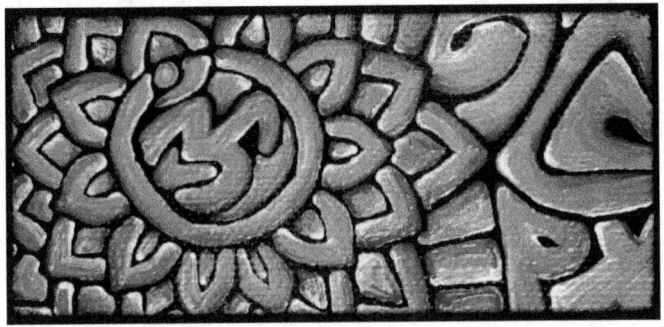

Sanskrit Name: Sahsrara (meaning thousand-fold)

Colour: Violet, gold, white (or a combination)

Location: Top of head

Corresponding areas: Spirituality, bliss, enlightenment, self-realization, spiritual connection, consciousness, claircognizance (clear knowing), divine guidance

Affirmation: I accept and honour the spirit within me and all living things.

Understanding the chakras helps us realize that everything really is connected. As we become more aware of how mind, body and spirit are intertwined, we can take more conscious steps to heal and harmonize every part of our selves and our lives. Plus, now you might just know what your yoga teacher means when she asks you to "let your anahata unfold!"

CHAPTER THREE

IMPORTANCE OF BREATHING AND BREATHING TECHNIQUE

➤ **Breathing makes you calmer.** Breathing deeply and feeling calm is your natural state. Deep breathing naturally relaxes the mind and body. Breathing deeply is the fastest way to stimulate the parasympathetic nervous system, aka the relaxation response, which makes you feel relaxed. Stress is at the core of most diseases and most of us live stressful busy lives, which is commonly accompanied with shallow breathing. When we breathe shallowly, the body does not receive as much oxygen as it needs and it makes our muscles constrict. You can almost feel this tightening when you are stressed or tense. The sympathetic nervous system is triggered when we feel stress or anxiety and sends out spikes of cortisol and adrenaline. It is the parasympathetic nervous system which counteracts this and breath is the fastest way for these two systems to communicate. With deeper breathing you can turn the switch from high alarm to low in seconds. Remember if you ever feel anxious to breathe deeply. Pay attention and you can feel the peace coming in and the tension being released as you simply (but deeply) breathe in and out.

➢ **Breathing helps to detoxify the body.** Our bodies are designed to release 70 percent of its toxins through breathing. Carbon dioxide is a natural toxic waste that comes from the body's metabolic processes and it needs to be expelled from the body regularly and consistently. It gets transferred from the blood to our lungs and we expel it with our breath. However, when our lungs are compromised by shallow breathing, the other detoxification systems in the body take over and have to work harder to expel this waste. This overload can make the body weaker and lead to illness.

➢ **Breathing relieves pain.** Studies have proved it yet when we feel pain our instant unconscious reaction is to hold our breath. Remember that breathing deeply and breathing into pain will help to release it. Deep breathing releases endorphins which are the body's natural feel good pain killers.

➢ **Breathing makes you happier.** Breathing deeply will increase the neurochemical production in the brain and release more of the ones that elevate moods and control pain.

➢ **Breathing helps to improve your posture.** Bad posture is often directly linked with incorrect breathing. Try it yourself and as you practise breathing deeply watch how you naturally straighten up. Filling your lungs encourages you to straighten your spine and stand or sit taller.

➢ **Breathing stimulates the lymphatic system.** The lymphatic system is a crucial system in our body that most of us are fairly unaware of. We know much more about our circulatory systems but we have twice the amount of lymphatic fluid in our body as we do blood. Our circulatory system relies on our heart to pump it, while the lymphatic system relies on our breathing to get it moving. The blood pumps oxygen and nutrients to the cells and once they absorb what they need they excrete their waste back out into the sea of lymphatic fluid that our cells constantly swim in. The lymph fluid is responsible for ridding the body of the debris the cells excrete and also dead cells and other waste. As our breathing is what moves the lymph, breathing shallowly can lead to a sluggish lymphatic system which is not detoxifying properly. Deep breathing will help get that lymph flowing properly so your body can work more efficiently.

➢ **Breathing increases our cardiovascular capacity.** It gives many of the same benefits of exercise and can enhance the benefits you get from exercise. Aerobic exercise (cardio) uses fat as energy, while anaerobic exercise (strength training) uses glucose as energy. By expanding our cardiovascular capacity from deep breathing we can do more cardio easier, which also increases our cardiovascular capacity and burns more fat cells as well.

➢ **Breathing gives you energy.** Drawing air deeper down into the lungs greatly increases blood flow as this is where the greatest amount of blood flow occurs, according to the American Medical Student Association. This increases energy and also improves stamina. The higher oxygen content of the blood, which cleanses the body and all its cells of debris and toxins, along with better circulation, better sleep, stress reduction, your body working more efficiently, and all that goes along with these naturally gives you lots more energy.

➢ **Breathing improves your digestion.** More oxygen is supplied to the digestive organs and thereby helping them to work more efficiently. Deeper breathing also results in an increased blood flow, which in the digestive tract encourages intestinal action and will further improve your overall digestion. It addition, deeper breathing results in a calmer nervous system which in turn also enhances optimal digestion.

➢ **Breathing strengthens the major organs of the body, such as lungs and the heart.** Deep breathing expands the lungs and makes them work more efficiently. It also brings in more oxygen to the blood which gets sent to the heart and makes it so that the heart does not have to work so hard to deliver oxygen to the tissues. Also, with the lungs working a little harder pushing out oxygen into the blood it eases the pressure needed by the heart to pump it through the body. This improves your circulation and gives the heart a bit of a break.

➤ **Breathing helps to regulate weight.** If you are underweight, the extra oxygen will help to feed the cells and tissues. If you are overweight it will assist with weight loss. The extra oxygen in the body will help to burn up excess fat more efficiently. When we are stressed, and most of us live day to day in a fairly stressed state, your body tends to burn glycogen instead of fat. Deep breathing triggers the relaxation response which encourages the body to burn fat instead.

DEEP BREATHING TECHNIQUES

Beyond the practice of simple deep breathing, the ancient yogis described different types of rhythmic deep breathing techniques that can have differing effects on the mind and body. In fact, many studies document the beneficial effects of yogic breathing in treating depression, anxiety, PTSD (posttraumatic stress disorder), COPD (chronic destructive pulmonary disease), and asthma.

There are also theories that support the notion that by slowing down and controlling the breath, we can improve our longevity.

The basis for all deep breathing practices originates in the science of yoga, specifically the branch of yoga known as pranayama. The word pranayama is derived from two Sanskrit words: prana (life force) and yama (control). By controlling the breath, you can influence every aspect of your life. You can train yourself to breathe in a way that has a positive influence on your health.

Each of the following simple yogic breathing techniques has specific effects on the mind-body physiology.

Complete Belly Breath: With one hand on your belly, relax your abdominal muscles, and slowly inhale through the nose, bringing air into the bottom of your lungs. You should feel your abdomen rise. This expands the lower parts of the lungs. Continue to inhale as your rib cage expands outward, and finally, the collar bones rise. At the peak of the inhalation, pause for a moment, then exhale gently from the top of your lungs to the bottom. At the end of exhalation, contract your abdominal muscles slightly to push residual air out of the bottom of your lungs.

Alternate Nostril Breathing: When you are feeling anxious or ungrounded, practice Alternate Nostril Breathing, known as Nadi Shodhana in the yogic tradition. This will immediately help you feel calmer.

- ➢ Hold your right thumb over your right nostril and inhale deeply through your left nostril.
- ➢ At the peak of your inhalation, close off your left nostril with your fourth finger, lift your right thumb, and then exhale smoothly through your right nostril.
- ➢ After a full exhalation, inhale through the right nostril, closing it off with your right thumb at the peak of your inhalation, lift your fourth finger and exhale smoothly through your left nostril.
- ➢ Continue with this practice for 3 to 5 minutes, alternating your breathing through each nostril. Your breathing should be effortless, with your mind gently observing the inflow and outflow of breath.

Ocean's Breath: When you feel angry, irritated, or frustrated, try a cooling pranayama such as Ocean's Breath, or Ujjayi (pronounced oo-jai). This will immediately soothe and settle your mind.

➤ Take an inhalation that is slightly deeper than normal. With your mouth closed, exhale through your nose while constricting your throat muscles. If you are doing this correctly, you should sound like waves on the ocean.

➤ Another way to get the hang of this practice is to try exhaling the sound "haaaaah" with your mouth open. Now make a similar sound with your mouth closed, feeling the outflow of air through your nasal passages.

➤ Once you have mastered this on the outflow, use the same method for the inflow breath, gently constricting your throat as you inhale.

Energizing Breath: When you are feeling blue or sluggish, try Energizing Breath or Bhastrika. This will give you an immediate surge of energy and invigorate your mind.

> ➤ Begin by relaxing your shoulders and take a few deep, full breaths from your abdomen.
> ➤ Now start exhaling forcefully through your nose, followed by forceful, deep inhalations at the rate of one second per cycle. Your breathing is entirely from your diaphragm, keeping your head, neck, shoulders, and chest relatively still while your belly moves in and out.
> ➤ Start by doing a round of ten breaths, then breathe naturally and notice the sensations in your body. After 15 to 30 seconds, begin the next round with 20 breaths. Finally, after pausing for another 30 seconds, complete a third round of 30 breaths. Beginners are advised to take a break between rounds.

Although Bhastrika is a safe practice, stay tuned in to your body during the process. If you feel light-headed or very uncomfortable, stop for a few moments before resuming in a less intense manner.

Contraindications: Do not practice Bhastrika if you are pregnant or have uncontrolled hypertension, epilepsy/seizures, panic disorder, hernia, gastric ulcer, glaucoma, or vertigo. Use caution if there is an underlying lung disease.

A regular daily practice of deep breathing is one of the best tools for improving your health and well-being. Performing one of these breath techni ues twice daily for only three to five minutes can produce long-term benefits.

You can also use them any time you are feeling stressed or notice that your breathing has become constricted. By training your body with a regular practice of deep breathing, you will begin to breathe more effectively even without concentrating on it.

CHAPTER FOUR

YOGA POSES

BOAT POSE / PARIPURNA NAVASANA

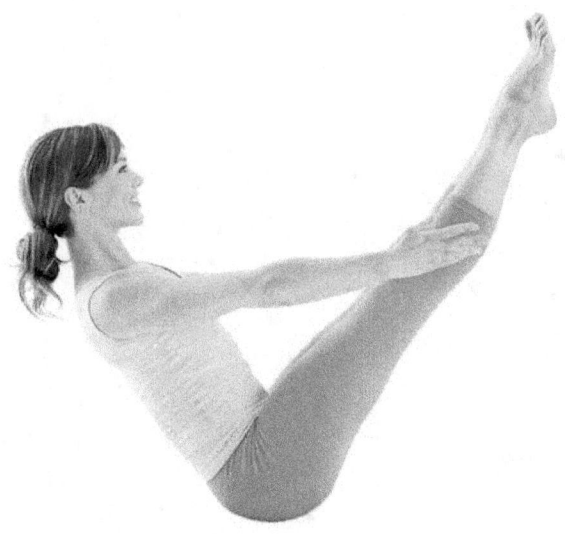

PROCEDURES

Take a seat together with your knees bent, feet on ground, arms behind you, arms pointing closer to the toes.

Make bigger the backbone, draw the stomach in and widen the collar bones to open the chest.

Lean lower back at the tripod among take a seat bones and sacrum and lift your feet off the floor, bringing the shins degree with the floor.

Preserving the increase through the backbone and preserve the chest open, fingers extend to the front parallel to the ground at the same time as viable straighten the legs out, nevertheless keeping the boost through the spine. Take 2-5 breaths, paintings up to ten breaths.

BENEFITS

  - ➢ Improves core strength
  - ➢ Strengthens the hip flexors and spine
  - ➢ Helps to relieve stress
  - ➢ Stimulates digestion

BRIDGE POSE / SETU BANDHA SARVANGASANA

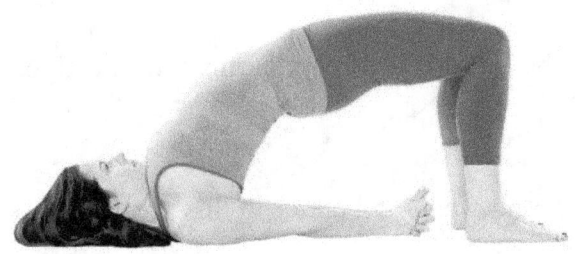

PROCEDURES

Lie on your back with your arms by the body, palms down.

Twist your knees and spot your feet level on the floor, heels near the rear end, hip width separated.

With the feet parallel to each other, press the upper arms into the floor, press your feet into the floor (inside and outside similarly) and start to lift the hips up to the roof, moving your breastbone to the jaw, yet not the button to the breastbone. Lift your jaw somewhat to hold space under the back of the neck.

Firm your tailbone towards the pubic bone and your pubic bone moves somewhat towards the paunch.

Effectively ac□uire the knees out front of you to hold the lower back amplified. Keep the knees over the lower legs.

Your rear end are firm yet not clenched. Your hips are lifted as high as is accessible to you with these standards set up.

Fasten your hands behind the back and firm the arms into the floor, shoulder bones are down along the spine.

You can take somewhere around 5 and 15 breaths in this posture.

To turn out, discharge the arms and let the hips down to the floor on an out-breath.

BENEFITS

- ➢ Stretches chest and spine.
- ➢ Strengthens legs, glutes and upper back.
- ➢ Improves digestion.
- ➢ Reduces backache and headache.
- ➢ Calms the mind, improves the mood.
- ➢ Can help to open the sinuses.

CAMEL POSE / USTRASANA

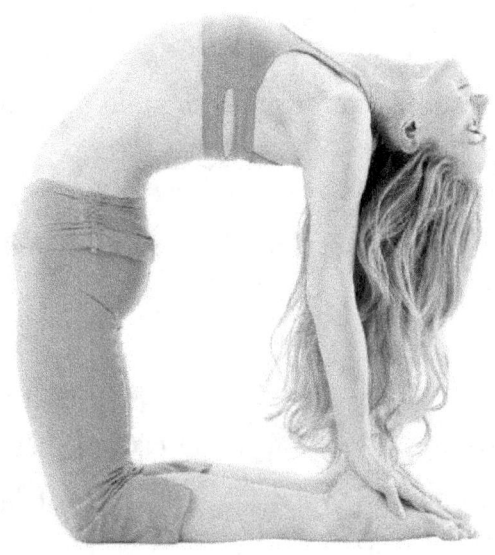

PROCEDURES

Gone ahead your knees, put the knees hip width separated, body upright. Toes tucked under, or on the off chance that you are more adaptable, point your toes back.

Place your hands on your lower back, heels of the hands laying on the lower back, fingers indicating down.

Connect with your legs. Pull the thighs back so the hips are still over the knees. Turn the inward thighs in a little and with your hands extend the bum down. In the meantime imagine drawing the front hipbones together and up to initiate the midsection. Your hip bones and lower ribs firm towards each other. Attempt to keep up this activity all through the posture.

With the lower body stable, start to take in towards the mid-section, moving the shoulder bones back as you lift the mid-section.

On a breathe out begin to come into your backbend keeping the mid-section lifted and without crunching the neck or lower back.

You can keep the head nonpartisan all through the posture, jaw towards the sternum (prescribed), in the event that you take the head back, do as such just when the opening in the mid-section is at its fullest and your neck is long and cheerful.

Lift the lower back ribs far from the lumbar spine to make considerably more length in the lower back and to encourage the opening in the mid-section much more.

Stay in this stance anywhere in the range of 30 seconds to a moment, breathing into the mid-section to encourage the opening there. When you see you can't inhale appropriately you are taking the posture too far and you ought to back off to a variety you can manage with breathing easily.

To turn out, spot the hands to the front hip bones and guide them down as you lift move down on an inward breath. In the event that your head is the distance back lead with the heart, bring the head up last. Kill and extend your spine in Downward Facing Dog Pose before resting in Child's Pose for a couple of breaths.

BENEFITS

> ➤ Opens the belly, chest, heart, shoulders and upper back.
> ➤ Stretches the whole front of the body including ankles, thighs and groin.
> ➤ Strengthens the legs and back.
> ➤ Improves your posture.
> ➤ Stimulates the organs in the belly.
> ➤ Energizes body and mind.

CAT POSE / MAJARYASANA

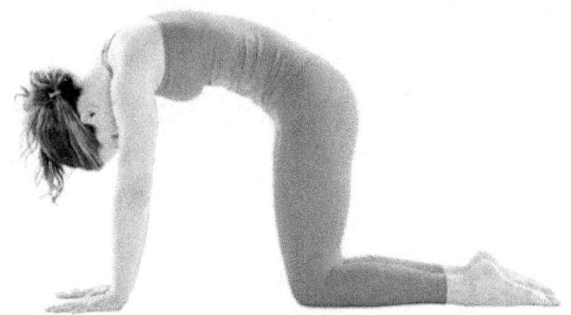

PROCEDURES

Begin staring you in the face and knees (all fours). Knees specifically under hips and wrists, elbows and shoulders in accordance with each other. Neck in accordance with your spine, look laying delicately on the floor.

Spread your fingers and press over the base of the fingers and the fingertips.

Breathe out and round your spine towards the roof, lifting the side abdomens.

Pull in your abs and tuck your tailbone, delicately getting your glutes. Attempt to keep your shoulders and knees in position.

Discharge your head towards the floor and press solidly into your hands.

Breathe in and return into your unbiased beginning position.

BENEFITS

> Stretches the back and neck.
> Gently massages the spine, increasing mobility.
> A great warm up before yoga practice.
> Helps relieve stress.
> Increases circulation of spinal fluid.
> Massages your digestive organs.
> Stimulates blood circulation in the wrists, especially helpful after a lot of computer work.

FISH POSE / MATSYASANA

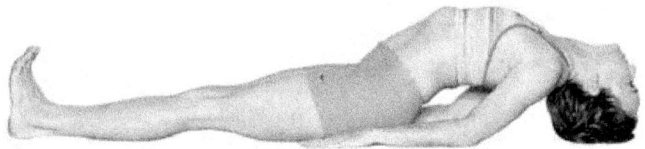

PROCEDURES

Rests on your back, curve your knees with the soles of your feet on the floor, arms nearby the body, palms down.

Raise your hips and slide your hands underneath the upper rump. Keep your gluteus muscles linked with your hands all through this stance.

Breathe in and press into your elbows and shoulders, lifting the mid-section.

Contingent upon the force of your back twist, either the back or the highest point of the head is on the floor. However there ought to be almost no weight on it.

On the off chance that this feels stable develop one leg out along the floor at once. Reach out through the heels, with a slight internal pivot of the upper legs.

Inhale, hold the posture for around 5 breaths.

Leave this posture when you are prepared by s□ueezing in the elbows, lifting the head back off the floor and slide the head down.

BENEFITS

- ➢ Energizing.
- ➢ Stretches the chest and intercostal muscles between the ribs.
- ➢ Opens and stimulates the neck, belly and its organs.
- ➢ Improves □uality of your breath.
- ➢ Counterpose for Shoulderstand.

EASY POSE / SUKHASANA

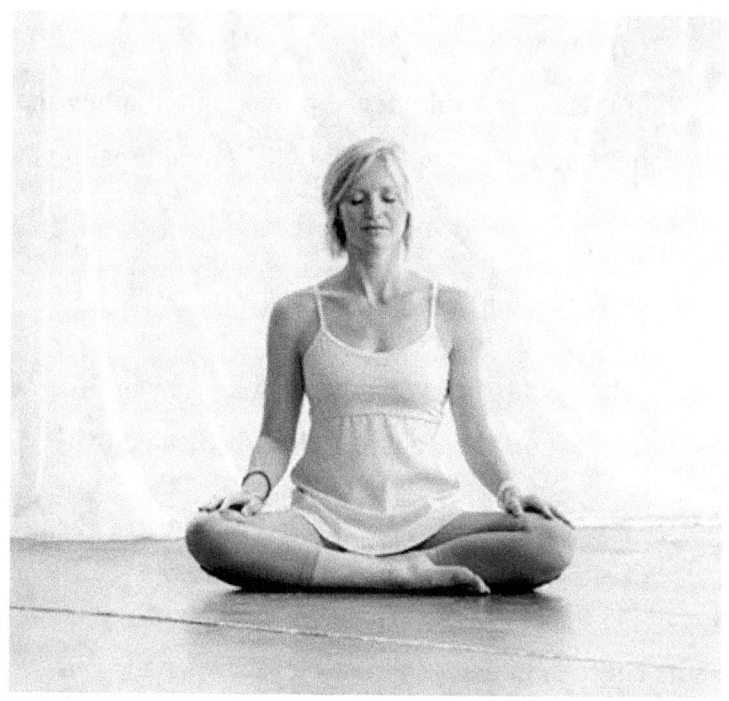

PROCEDURES

Start sitting on the mat with the sit-bones on the front edge of a firm pad or collapsed cover.

Cross your shins parallel to the mat, bringing every foot underneath the inverse knee. Attempt to align your feet with the knees.

Extend your spine keeping the characteristic curves in the spine, push the sit bones into the floor to root down and make length through the crown of your head. Firm your shoulder bones in.

Place your hands on your lap or knees with palms up (more open), or palms down (Quieting).

Attempt to switch the cross of your legs when you next come into the stance.

BENEFITS

- ➢ Calms the mind
- ➢ Strengthens the back
- ➢ Opens your hips
- ➢ Good preparation for meditation or for Pranayama

GATE POSE / PARIGHASANA

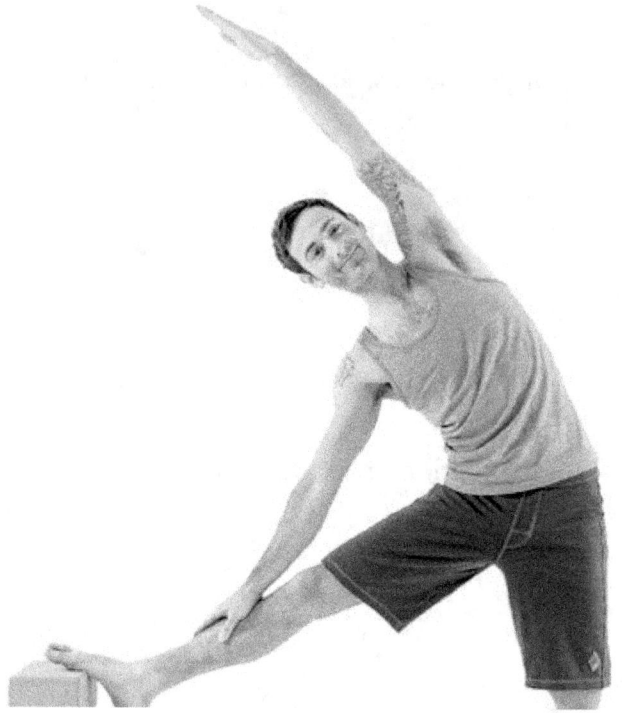

PROCEDURES

Stoop on the mat, confronting the long side of your mat. Stretch your forgot leg and remotely turn the leg so that your heel rest on the mat with your knee and toes (foot flexed) indicating up. Turn your right hip marginally forward contrasted with the left hip. Keep the middle confronting the inside, even somewhat to one side open your arms out to the side parallel to the floor, palms confronting up. Breathe in, extend the body and breathe out, lower the left half of the body to left leg, setting the hand down on the left leg.

Ground through the right knee.

On an in-breath lift your right arm up and over to one side. Urge the right hip to continue moving forward a bit while in the meantime opening the middle to one side, looking under the right arm to the roof.

Stay in this posture between the 5-10 breaths. To turn out, breathe in reaching out through the top arm and return to focus.

Convey the knees back alongside each other and rehash on the opposite side.

BENEFITS

> Stretches the calves, hamstrings, spine.
> Opens the side body, chest and shoulders.
> Stimulates the lungs and the abdominal organs.
> Great for managing your love handles!
> Great for your balance.

HALF FROG POSE / ARDHA BHEKASANA

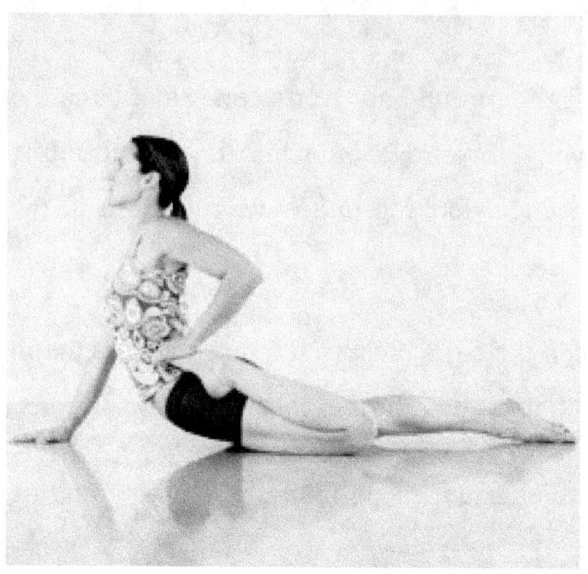

PROCEDURES

Lie on your stomach, on the lower arms, elbows underneath the shoulders.

Firm the pubic bone down and attract your tummy.

Cross the left lower arm before the body. Twist your right knee and compass back with the right hand to hold the highest point of your foot, pulling the foot in towards the outside of your right hip.

Diminish the highest point of the right thigh, move the fingers towards the front if conceivable, turn the right side body towards the front too.

Stay associated with the breath.

Stay for 5 breaths before discharging the foot and gradually bringing it down to the ground.

Rehash with the other leg.

BENEFITS

- ➢ Stretches the thigh muscles and hip flexors.
- ➢ Increases the flexibility in the back.
- ➢ Opens the chest and shoulders.
- ➢ Stimulates your energy.
- ➢ Prepares the body for back bending.
- ➢ Great stretch for runners and cyclists.

HAPPY BABY POSE / ANANDA BALASANA

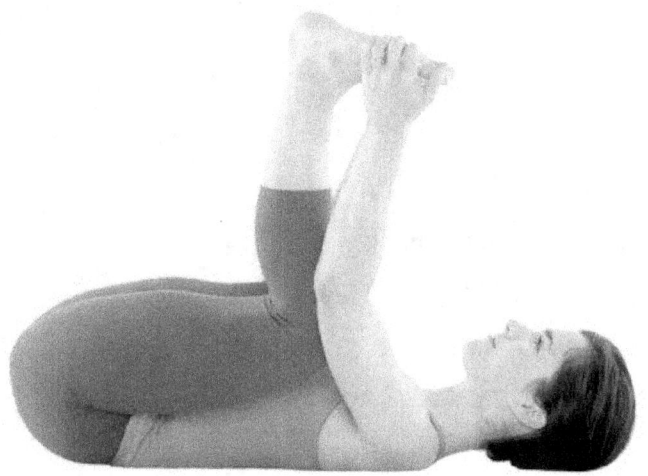

PROCEDURES

Lie on your back with your knees bowed into your mid-section.

Breathe in - get the outside of your feet.

Open your knees more extensive than your middle and convey them towards the floor alongside the armpits.

Ensure your lower leg is specifically over your knees (90 degree point).

Flex through your heels, tenderly pushing your feet into your hands, pulling the hands down to make resistance.

Attempt to acquire thighs towards the middle and down towards the floor.

Augment your spine by protracting your tailbone and draw your gut marginally in.

Keep up the length in the back of your neck.

Hold for 30 - 60 seconds.

To leave the posture, bring feet back onto the floor on a breathe out.

BENEFITS

> Gently stretches inner groin and spine.
> Calms the mind, relieving stress and fatigue.
> Opens hips.
> Strengthens the arms.
> Releases and decompresses the sacroiliac joint.

HEAD TO KNEE POSE / JANU SIRSASANA

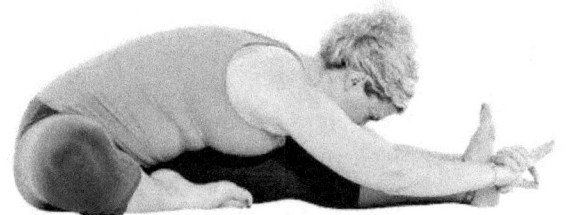

PROCEDURES

Sit with the legs outstretched before you (Staff Pose/Dandasana).

Breathe in twist your right knee and spot the right foot against the left internal thigh, breathe out let the right knee lay on (or towards) the floor.

Flex the left foot, press the highest point of the thigh down, extend the spine on an in-breath and on an out-breath turn the spine a little to confront the left leg and afterward overlap forward from the hips.

Keep your spine long, mid-section open and shoulders drawn down. Unwind your face.

Grab hold of your foot, lower leg or wherever your hands reach on your leg. In the event that your hands come past your foot you can grab hold of the right wrist with the left hand and tie around the left foot

Stay in the stance for 5 to 10 breaths.

Breathe in to leave the posture.

BENEFITS

- ➤ Calms the mind and is therapeutic for mild depression.
- ➤ Stimulates digestion.
- ➤ Stretches the hips, back of the body and groins.
- ➤ Relieves menstrual discomfort, headache, anxiety and fatigue.
- ➤ Stimulates the kidneys and liver.

HERON POSE / KROUNCHASANA

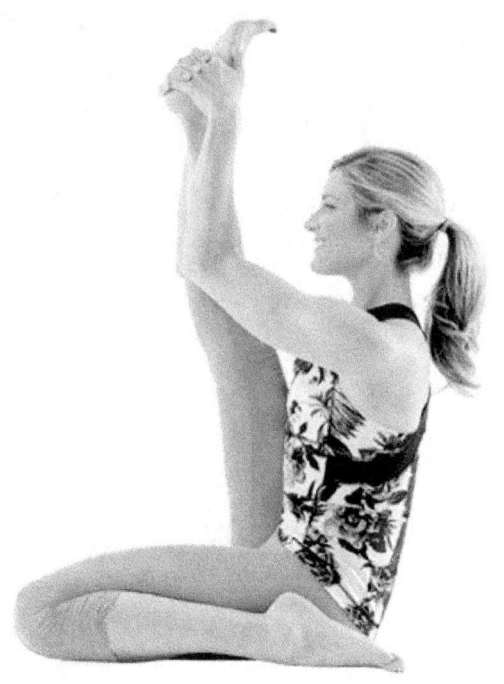

PROCEDURES

Sit in Dandasana, with your legs outstretched before you.

Breathe out curve your right knee and convey the foot alongside the right hip. So the highest point of the foot is on the floor and toes are indicating once again into Half Virasana Pose.

Ensure you are sitting equitably on both sit bones. You can utilize a piece or collapsed cover under both sit bones or the sit bone of the straight leg.

Twist your left leg, put the foot on the floor. Grab hold of the left foot with both hands.

Keep the shoulder bones firm on the back, to keep the mid-section open. On an inward breath start to rectify your left leg, while keeping the spine long, mid-section open and the sternum lifted.

Once the leg is straight, breathe out and acquire the leg near the mid-section. In the event that you can keep up all the past activities guide the head towards the shin bone.

Hold for around 5 breaths and discharge the leg on an exhalation and return into Dandasana.

BENEFITS

> ➢ Stretches the bent leg thigh, ankle and shin.
> ➢ Stretches the back of the straight leg, including the Achilles tendon.
> ➢ Improves core stability.

HERO POSE / VIRASANA

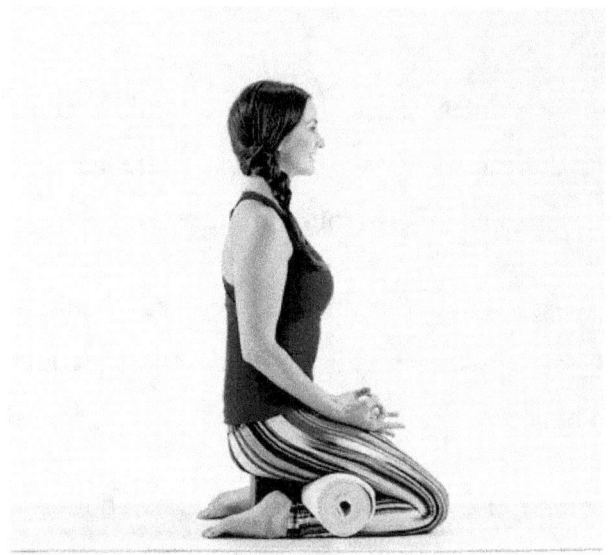

PROCEDURES

Begin by staring your face and knees with your knees specifically under your hips

Unite your knees and your feet somewhat more extensive than hip width

Press the highest points of the feet immovably into the mat

Begin to bring down your hips back gradually with the goal that you are in the long run sitting on the mat (or props) between your heels - you may need to roll the substance of the calves away

Continue checking in with your knees the entire time while coming into the posture to ensure there are no sharp or curving sensations.

For some individuals sitting onto the heels or setting a s□uare or pad between the heels to sit on will be more secure for the knees and less demanding for the □uadriceps.

Hold the toes indicating back and the inward lower legs attracted ensure the knees

Attract your navel and up, protract your tailbone to the floor and reach out through the crown of your head

Stay in the stance for 5 to 10 breaths

Left the represent the way you came in, by putting the hands before you and lifting the hips move down to a tabletop (all fours) position or by moving your base over to the other side with the goal that you can develop one leg then the other into Dandasana

You can likewise stay in Virasana for more periods and use it as a posture for reflection. For this situation it is more agreeable for a great many people to utilize props (pieces or pads) to sit on.

BENEFITS

- ➢ Stretches ankles, tops of the feet, knees, and legs
- ➢ Calming
- ➢ Energises the legs when they are tired
- ➢ A great alternative to Lotus pose for meditation

LOCUST POSE / SALABHASANA

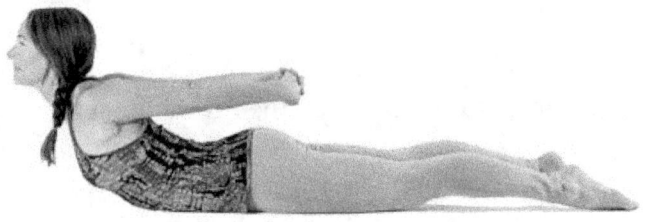

PROCEDURES

Lie on your stomach, arms close by, palms confronting down, the front of your button is on the floor.

Extend your lower back by delicately s ueezing your pubic bone into the floor, and draw your navel in towards the spine as you breathe out.

Draw in your leg muscles.

Breathe in lift your head, mid-section, arms and legs off the floor, firming your shoulder bones onto your back, thus opening your heart. You can envision somebody holding your hands and pulling you back, to come up higher.

Feet are drawn towards the mid-line however don't need to touch, you can keep them hip-width separated.

Hold the stance for 5 breaths ensuring breathing stays cool and unfaltering.

Breathe out to bring down out of the stance then rehash another two times.

Rest in the middle of every posture by making a pad for your cheek with your arms and giving your heels a chance to drop far from each other.

BENEFITS

> Improves strength and flexibility in the back muscles.
> Stretches the front of the body.
> Improves stamina.
> Opens the chest.
> Stimulates the abdominal organs.

LOTUS POSE / PADMASANA

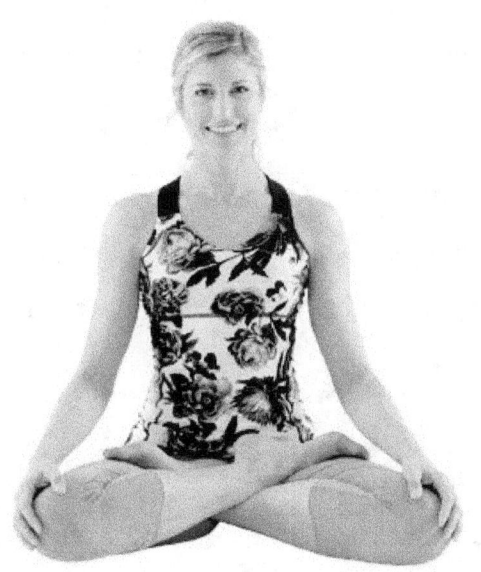

PROCEDURES

From a situated with folded legs position, ground the hips. Breathe in and protract through the spine.

Take the right foot in the elbow wrinkle of the left arm and the knee in the right elbow or hand.

Support the lower leg to relax out the hip joint and investigate its scope of movement. At the same time keeping the spine straight.

Breathe out, bring the right leg as far out to the great, close the knee by uniting thigh and calf.

At that point breathe in and bring the outside of the right foot to rest in the inward left crotch. Guarantee the turn originates from the hip and not the knee joint.

Presently get the left leg. Rehash the activities of supporting the leg to relax the hip and shutting the knee. Turn the leg from the hip and slide the left leg over the privilege with your left foot into the right crotch.

Draw the knees as near one another as could be expected under the circumstances.

Convey the backs of your hands to the knees with your fingers in Jnana mudra - thumbs and first fingers touching.

Keep the spine long and the look to the floor in front of you.

Stay in the posture for 10 breaths or more. Left the represent the converse way you came in by uncrossing one leg deliberately and afterward the following. Begin with the left foot next time.

BENEFITS

- ➤ Increases flexibility in the hips.
- ➤ Calms the brain.
- ➤ Used for Pranayama practice.

LORD OF THE DANCE POSE / NATARAJASANA

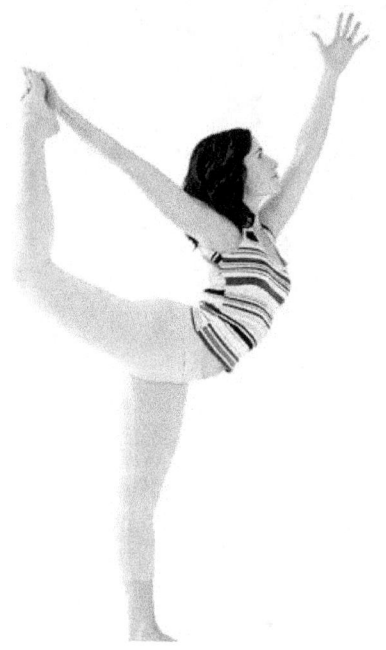

PROCEDURES

Stand in Tadasana. Ground and focus through your feet and take a point on eye level to concentrate on. Breathe out curve your left knee, left foot to the butt cheek, and hold the outside of your left foot with the left hand. The highest point of the right thighbone steps back and connect with your right thigh and knee to make the standing leg solid.

Keep the middle upright, the mid-section open and attract the pubic issue that remains to be worked out navel to keep length in the lower back. Presently on a breathe in pushing the left foot once more into the hand, raising the leg so the thighbone winds up parallel to the floor and the lower leg in a right edge with the thigh bone and vertical with the floor. You can lift your right arm up before you, parallel to the floor or somewhat higher by the ear.

Hold for 5-10 breaths.

On an out-breath discharge the leg withdraw to the floor.

BENEFITS

> ➤ Strengthens the ankles, legs, core and arms.
> ➤ Stretches the chest, shoulders, groins and abdomen.
> ➤ Improves balance and concentration.

TREE POSE / VRKSASANA

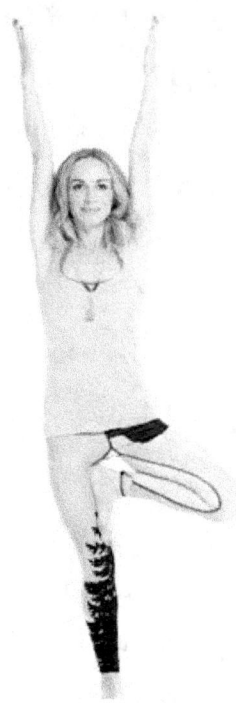

PROCEDURES

From Mountain posture, move your weight on to one side leg. Ground your left foot down into the floor, pull up your knee top and thigh.

Look at a point on eye level, to help you adjust.

Twist your right knee, reach down with your right hand and fasten your lower leg.

With help of the hand, put your right foot within the left leg, if its accessible to you on the internal thigh, with your heel up high. Stretch your tailbone toward the floor.

On the off chance that that is not accessible to you, put within the foot within the lower leg or calf. Evade within the knee.

Twist the knee out to the side, press your foot against the inward thigh, and the internal thigh once more into the foot.

Ac□uire your hands front of your heart in petition position, or you can lift your arms up to the roof. hands shoulder width separated.

With arms lifted, lift from the back body.

Stay in this stance for around 30 sec or 1 min.

On an outbreath bring down the leg and arms down and remain in Tadasana, rehash on the opposite side.

BENEFITS

> Stretches the spine, shoulders and back of the legs.
> Opens the upper back and chest.
> Balances the thyroid gland.
> Stimulates the abdominal organs.

- Calms the mind and reduces stress and fatigue.
- Therapeutic for sinusitis, infertility and insomnia.
- Relieves backpain and headaches.

PLOW POSE / HALASANA

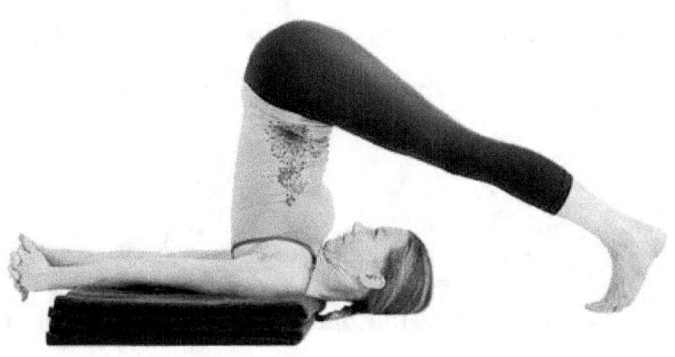

PROCEDURES

From Salamba Sarvangasana bring down the feet to the floor pivoting from the hips.

On the other hand lie on your back with your upper back on a durable collapsed cover, your head is laying on the mat, so the sweeping closures in the empty of the neck. The capacity of the cover is to diminish the stretch in the back of the neck, to hold the back of the neck from smoothing excessively. You may re□uire more than one cover - ensure they are perfectly collapsed and stacked.

Breathe out draw your lower paunch into your spine and firm it once again into the floor.

Press your arms into the floor, breathe in and lift your legs over your head towards the floor.

Permit the feet to bring down towards the floor, maybe the toes achieve the floor, tuck the toes on the off chance that they do. Stretch out through the heels.

Keep your look turning upward, head still, confront loose.

Augment your arms out, intertwine the hands, walk your shoulders towards each other, with the expectation to open the mid-section. Firming the upper back to the mid-section too.

With an open mid-section, keeping your button somewhat up to keep the throat delicate, place your hands on your lower back to bolster yourself.

Discover the lift of the spine from the establishing through the arms and shoulders, and feet on the off chance that they are on the floor.

Tailbone spans to the roof, hips over shoulders, keeping the spine long and lift the highest point of the thighs. Stay here for 5 to 10 breaths. To leave the posture, essentially discharge your hands and take your arms back to parallel on the floor by you, palms down and take off of the stance on a breathe out.

BENEFITS

> ➤ Improves balance
> ➤ Opens the hips
> ➤ Strengthens the ankles, legs and spine
> ➤ Lengthens the spine
> ➤ Improves focus or concentration

CHAPTER FIVE

THE BEST YOGA WORKOUT FOR BEGINNERS

Yoga works great for helping you relax and focus, but it's also great for increasing your flexibility and helping to build strength.

If you're limited on time each morning, we've got a great yoga routine that only takes a few minutes each day, and won't leave you worn out before you head out of the house.

YOGA WORKOUT ROUTINE

Get Warmed Up

Warrior II (Virabhadrasana II)

Reverse Warrior (Viparita Virabhadrasana)

Cow Pose (Bitilasana)

Cat Pose (Marjaryasana)

Downward Dog (Adho Mukha Svanasana)

Extended Side Angle (Utthita Parsvakonasana)

Locust Pose (Salabhasana)

Corpse Pose (Savasana)

To get the most out of this routine, you will want to flow through each pose two different times, until you finally end with the Corpse pose, or savasana. You'll only perform the corpse pose once, as it's may focus is to help you center for your day.

Get Warmed Up

Before you begin your routine, get your mat ready, and make sure you're in comfortable clothing that will bend and move with you, without making your body heat up too much.

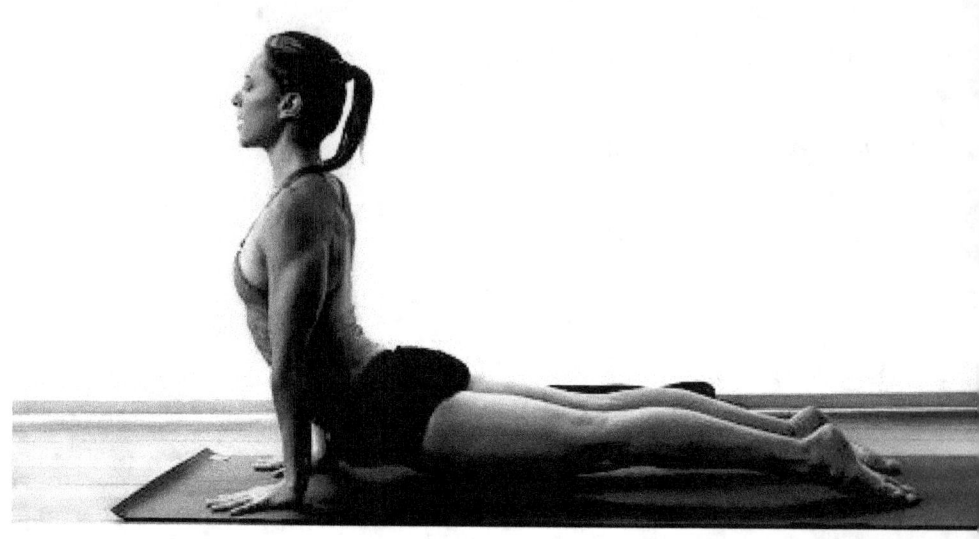

Then, sit down on the floor with your legs crossed in front of you. Begin by closing your eyes and breathing deep through your nose. Finish by exhaling through your mouth.

Bend over from side to side, breathing in as you lean down, and breathing out as you lean up to switch sides.

You should warm up for at least 5 to 10 minutes before you begin your poses, to prevent the risk of injury.

Warrior II (Virabhadrasana II)

To begin warrior pose, start with one foot in front of you and the other behind you, with your heels spread 3 to 4 feet apart, one in front of you, and one behind you. Stiffen your thighs, and turn your left leg out so that your knee cap is in line with your ankle.

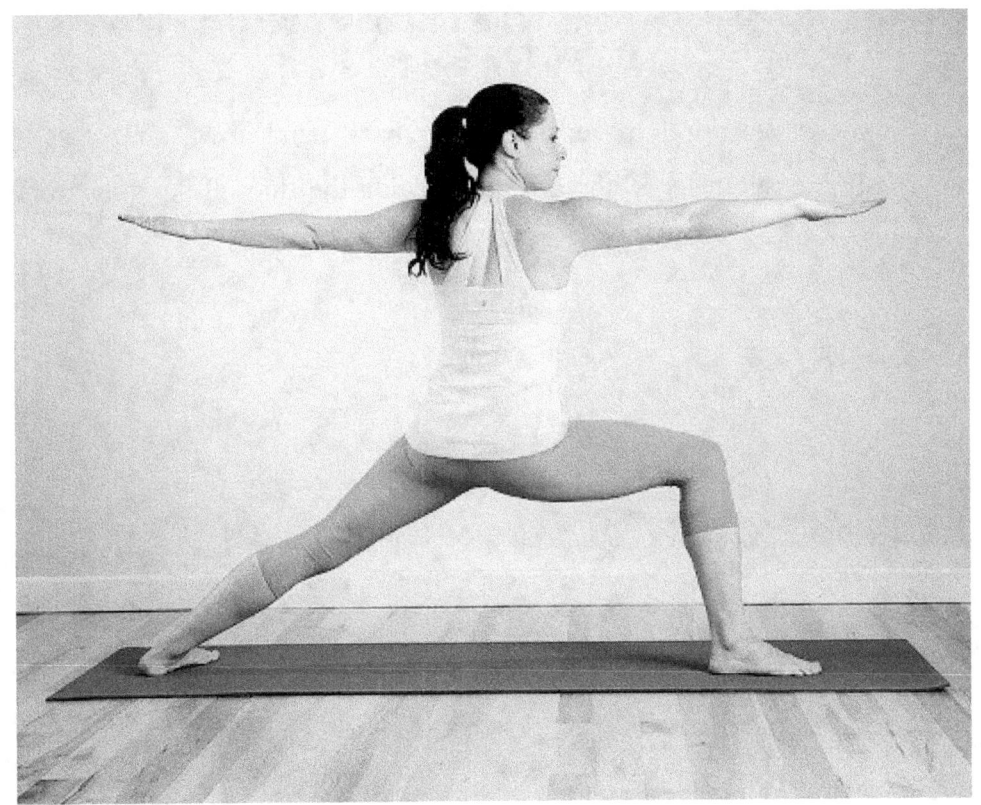

Then, exhale and bend your left knee over your left ankle. Now, apply pressure to your right leg, pressing your heel into the floor. Stretch your arms so you're creating space in your shoulders, while keeping your torso straight up and down.

Push your tailbone in, and then turn your head to the left, staring past your fingertips.

Reverse Warrior (Viparita Virabhadrasana)

From the Warrior II pose, bring your back hand down and plant it firmly onto your leg with your palm facing the floor. Take your front palm and face it towards the ceiling.

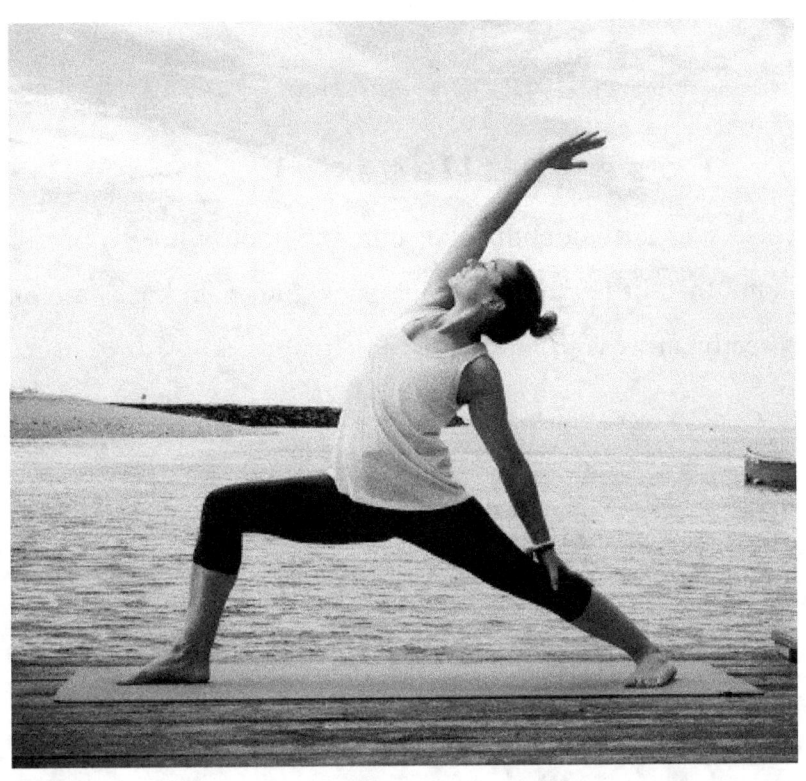

While inhaling, extend your front arm upwards, with your palm facing behind you. Focus on keeping your hips open, while pushing your chest towards the ceiling and your eyes pointing up.

Push the pose onto your front knee while you're stretching out your back leg.

Cow Pose (Bitilasana)

From Reverse Warrior, put both hands onto the floor in line with your shoulders, and then bring your front leg back until both knees are on the floor directly under your hips.

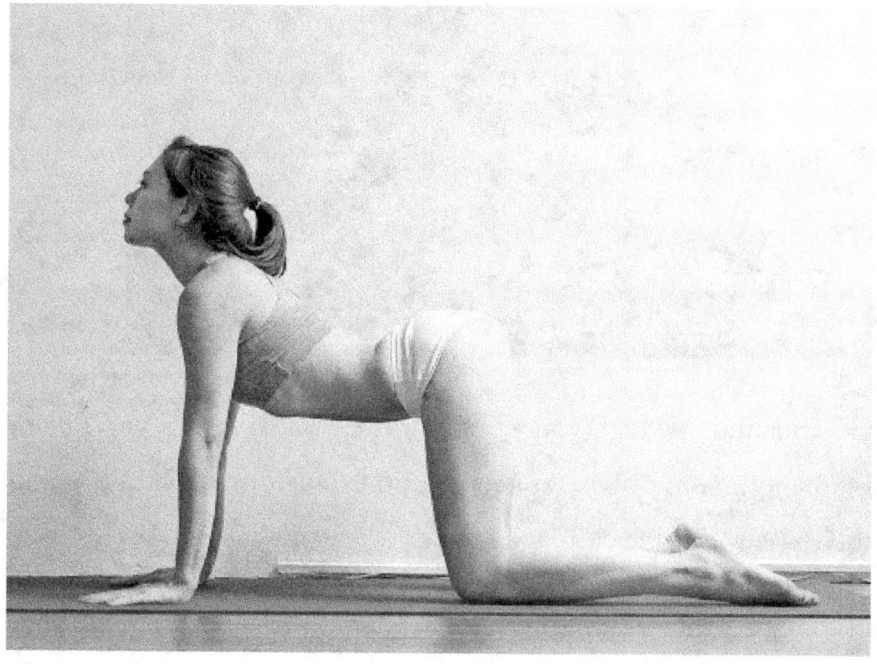

Now, inhale and lift your tailbone and chest upwards while pushing your belly down to the floor. Keep your head up, looking directly forward at the wall.

Cat Pose (Marjaryasana)

From the Reverse Warrior pose, exhale and push your spine upwards toward the ceiling. Make sure that you're keeping your shoulders above your hands, and your hips above your knees.

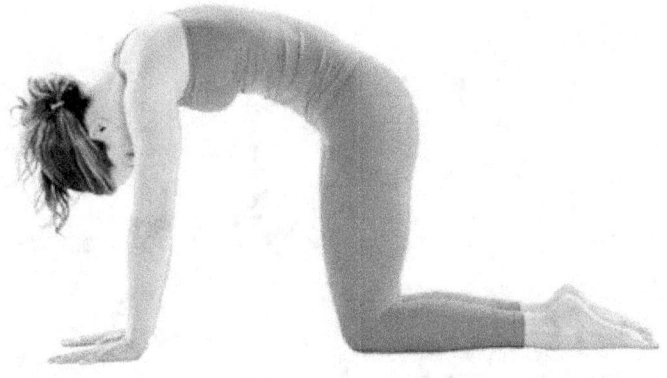

As you're pushing your spine upwards, you want to inhale and bring your body back to the cow pose, ensuring that you stay focused on your breathing while keeping your hips and shoulders open.

Downward Dog (Adho Mukha Svanasana)

From the Cat Pose, lift your knees from the floor, and begin pushing backwards onto your heels while keeping your hands flat against your mat.

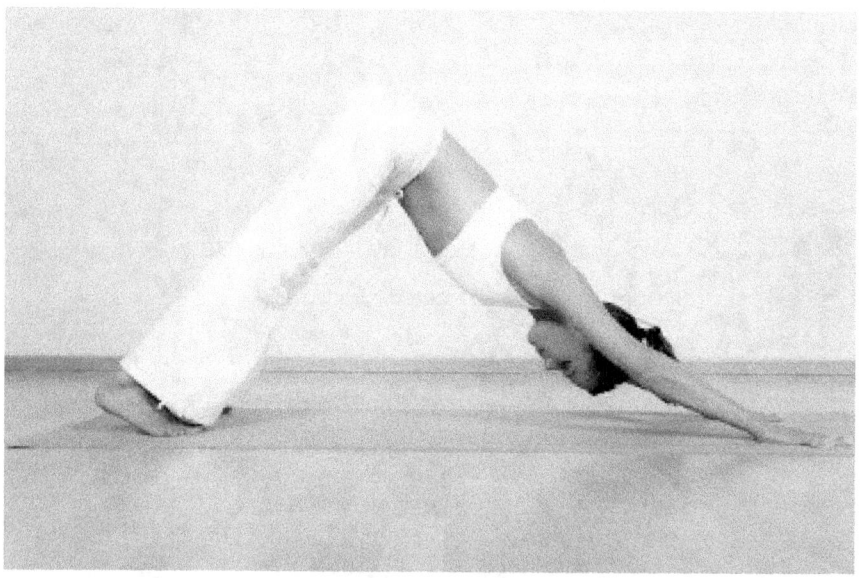

Work on aligning your arms and wrists with your hips, and keep the same angle with from your hips down to your heels. You're going to make an inverted "V" shape when you've got the right techni□ue.

Exhale while pushing your knees off of the floor, pushing your tailbone upwards and extending your legs downwards onto your toes. Remember not to lock your knees.

As you're pushing your toes down into the floor, you also want to push your hands into the floor in front of you. Hold the pose as you inhale and exhale multiple times.

Extended Side Angle (Utthita Parsvakonasana)

From Downward Dog, extend your left leg out in front of you, 3 to 4 feet away from your right foot. Turn your left foot out while pointing your right foot directly forward, keeping your heels aligned.

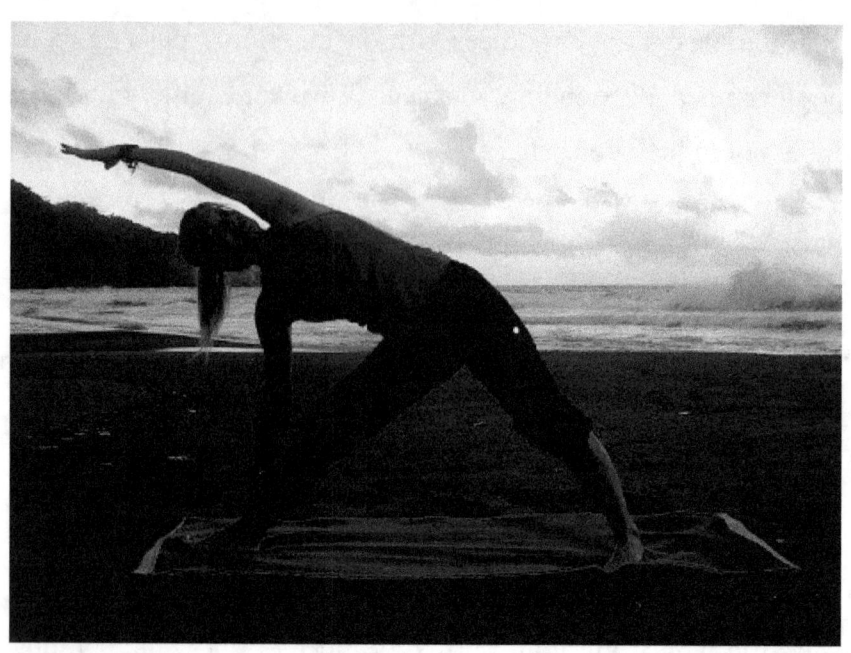

Now, lift your groin into your pelvis, and then breathe out as you bend over your right foot until your thigh is even with the floor beneath you.

Push down into your left heel and reach your right hand towards the ceiling while your left hand grabs onto the top of your right foot. Push your right knee into your left arm as you're twisting your body, pushing your chest out.

Locust Pose (Salabhasana)

From Extended Side Angle, push both feet out behind you and then lay down on the floor with your belly touching the mat. Push your arms down the sides of your torso, and turn your toes in towards each other.

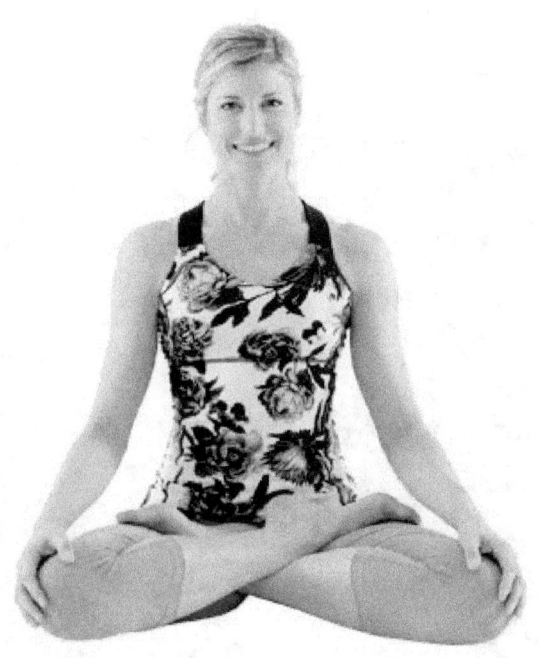

Firm up your butt while pushing your pelvis into the floor, then exhale and lift your upper torso, arms, legs, and head. Reach down through your legs with your arms, locking your hands together behind your back and tailbone.

Continue lifting your head from the floor, while using your locked hands to stretch backwards towards your feet. Then, push your feet through the floor, extending your hips, thighs, and calves.

Corpse Pose (Savasana)

From the Locust Pose, release and roll over to your back. This pose is to help you gain clarity and recenter your body and mind.

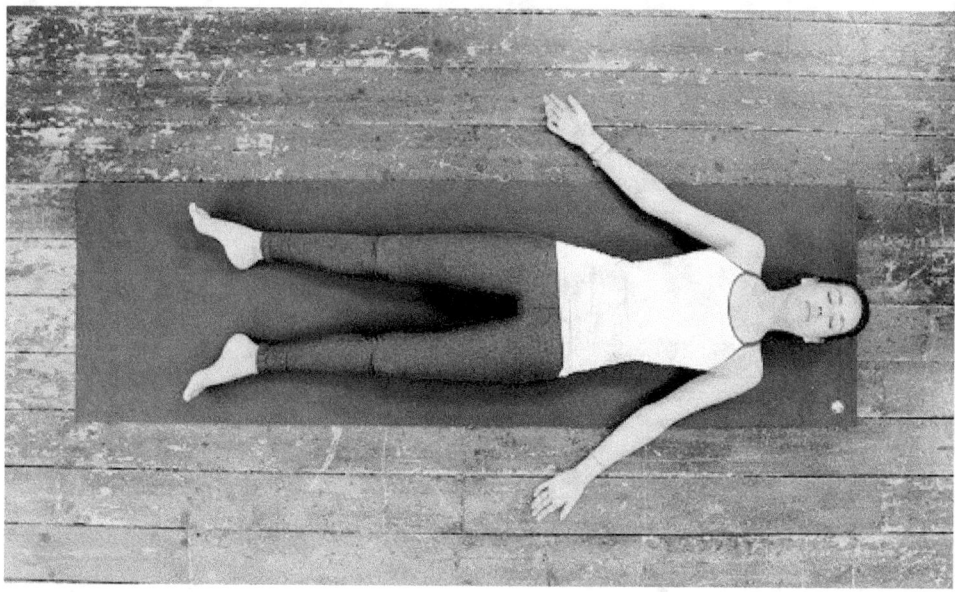

While laying on your back, lift the base of your neck so that your head is resting, pushing back and pointing your eyes towards the ceiling behind you.

Take your arms and lay them softly on the mat next to you, with your palms facing upwards, relaxing your fingers.

Then, soften your pelvis and tailbone, allowing them to sink into the mat beneath you. Push your legs out, and then let them relax in front of you, keeping your knees the same distance apart as your shoulder blades.

You're going to want to hold this pose for at least 5 minutes, for every 30 minutes of your routine. Since this is a shorter routine focused on getting your day started, you only need to hold it for 5 minutes.

While you're in the corpse pose, focus on your breathing, and when you're finished, begin by pulling your legs off of the mat, followed by your pelvis, and then your upper body. Finish by slowly dragging your head off of the mat.

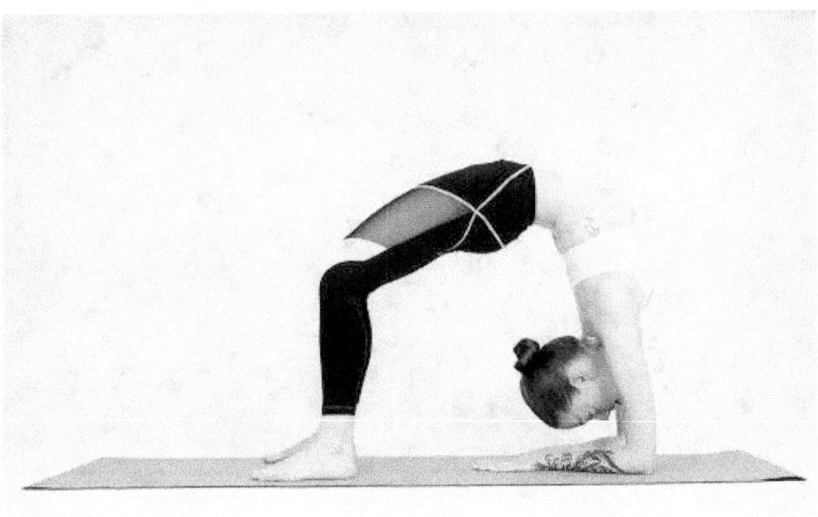

When you've finished completing this routine, be mindful about how you're feeling, and then pay attention to the thoughts you're having about the world as you progress through your daily life. If you notice yourself having negative thoughts or actions, try to correct your course, and then get down on the mat again if you have to.

Practicing a couple times per week is more than sufficient as you're just getting started, and you'll naturally want to increase how often you do yoga as you get a few sessions under your belt.

CONCLUSION

Yoga combines several techni ues to combat stress. Yoga provides a combination of benefits such as breathing exercises, stretching exercises, fitness programs, meditation practice and guided meditations all in one technique. That is powerful, very powerful! Even for people who have physical limitations yoga can be very beneficial just by practicing the breathing techni ues, the meditation and the guided meditation. Just by doing this you can have great benefits with the practice of yoga. So in conclusion yes, yoga can be a great remedy and highly effective for relieving stress. Yoga has combined set of principles and exercises that can greatly benefit you and help you to deal with stress in all forms.

www.ingramcontent.com/pod-product-compliance
Lightning Source LLC
Chambersburg PA
CBHW060152290526
45789CB00003B/1016